HIGH PERFORMANCE HEALTH
WORKBOOK

HIGH PERFORMANCE HEALTH
WORKBOOK

JAMES M. RIPPE, M.D.

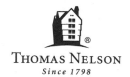

THOMAS NELSON
Since 1798

NASHVILLE DALLAS MEXICO CITY RIO DE JANEIRO BEIJING

Published in Nashville, Tennessee, by Thomas Nelson. Thomas Nelson is a trademark of Thomas Nelson, Inc.

Published in association with the literary agency of Alive Communications, Inc., 7680 Goddard St., Suite 200, Colorado Springs, CO 80920

Thomas Nelson, Inc. books may be purchased in bulk for educational, business, fund-raising, or sales promotional use. For information, please e-mail SpecialMarkets@ThomasNelson.com.

General Editor, Florida Hospital: Todd Chobotar
Florida Hospital Review Board: Alex Mattison, Stephanie Rick, Lillian Boyd
Photography: Spencer Freeman
Cover Design: Gearbox
Interior Design: Casey Hooper

Publishers Note: This book is not intended to replace a one-on-one relationship with a qualified healthcare professional but is in tended as a sharing of knowledge and information from the research and experience of the author. You are advised and encouraged to consult with your healthcare professional in all matters relating to your health and the health of your family. The publisher and author disclaim any liability arising directly or indirectly from the use of this book.

ISBN 978-1-4185-1979-7

Printed in the United States of America
1 2 3 4 5 6 RRD 10 09 08

To Stephanie, Hart, Jaelin, Devon, and Jamie,
who give my life meaning and purpose
and fill my heart with joy.

ACKNOWLEDGEMENTS

The concepts outlined in this book represent the work of many people over many years. While these individuals are too numerous to acknowledge all by name, I would like to particularly thank some key individuals who have led much of this effort.

Much of the research that forms the basis of this book and its companion book, *High Performance Health*, was performed at Rippe Lifestyle Institute and Rippe Lifestyle Institute of Florida under the able direction of my great friend and colleague Ted Angelopoulos, Ph.D., MPH. He is ably assisted by Linda Zukley, Ph.D., CCRN, who serves as the Associate Director of Research at RLI. Ted and Linda lead a large group of extremely dedicated and energetic exercise physiologists, nutritionists, nurses, physicians, and support personnel who conduct world class research every day.

A number of the clinical insights, which form the basis for this book as well as *High Performance Health*, come from my clinical facility, Rippe Health Assessment at Florida Hospital Celebration Health. The clinical team at RHA is led by Drs. Sherry Brooks, Sheri Novenstern, and Christine Edwards, as well as our Clinic Director, Herminio Alamo, MHA, RN. The clinicians who deliver great patient care every day at Rippe Health Assessment have provided key insights that led to the formulation many of the concepts in this workbook.

I have also been blessed to lead an academic effort at the University of Central Florida to establish the Center for Lifestyle Medicine at UCF. This would not have been possible without the strong support of the President of UCF, my friend and colleague Dr. John Hitt and the Provost of UCF, Dr. Terry Hickey.

The wonderful editorial team at Thomas Nelson, under the direction of Pamela Clements, has supported this and many other writing projects over the last two years. I would also like to acknowledge and thank my literary agent for this project, Lee Hough, who always provides great help and insight. Todd Chobotar, Director of Publishing and Creative Projects at Florida Hospital, has provided support and advice.

All of my writing projects are directed by my superb Editorial Director, Elizabeth Grady, who continues to amaze me with her organizational skills, good humor, and competence. Mary Abbott Waite, Ph.D., provided excellent editorial help on my previous book, *High Performance Health*, upon which this workbook is based. I would also like to particularly thank and acknowledge the excellent editorial work performed on the workbook manuscript by Steve Halliday.

My executive assistant, Carol Moreau, helps create time for these projects by managing my complex schedule. Carol does this with a very high level of caring, performance, and skill. Becky Cotton Hess, my executive assistant at Rippe Lifestyle Institute of Florida, performs similar duties flawlessly in Florida. My assistant at the University of Central Florida and coordinator for the Center for Lifestyle Medicine at UCF, Debbie Rhodes, also does a wonderful job.

I would also like to acknowledge and thank the thousand of patients and research subjects who have come through Rippe Lifestyle Institute and Rippe Health Assessment over the past two decades. Their stories and the insights that I have learned from working with them are peppered throughout this book.

Finally, I would like to acknowledge my dear wife, Stephanie Hart Rippe, who inspires me every day to be my best and to take time to stop and smell the roses as I juggle my way through a complex and busy life. She has been my soul mate and partner on this wonderful journey. Our four fantastic daughters, Hart, Jaelin, Devon, and Jamie continue to amaze me as they grow into wonderful young women. These five women together comprise the "Rippe Women" and bring more joy and meaning into my life than I ever thought possible.

JMR
Boston, MA

CONTENTS

INTRODUCTION

I have long been interested in what has been called *lifestyle medicine*—the dynamic link between actions and health. Why? It's simple, really.

First, an impressive body of medical literature insists that physical activity, good nutritional choices, effective weight management, and cessation of smoking all have a significant impact on health. At the same time, Americans eager for "miraculous" or "overnight" changes are turning to an exploding number of unproven and even dubious practices, all devoid of scientific proof.

Prodded by both my interest and concern, twenty years ago I established one of the first research laboratories and clinics in the world to focus on lifestyle medicine. In the years since, the clinic and its research arm have become the world leaders in the area of lifestyle medicine.

The Rippe Lifestyle Institute has presented and published more than three hundred academic papers on topics from stress reduction to nutrition, weight management, and fitness and their impact on disease prevention and management. In addition, the Rippe Health Assessment clinic at the Florida Hospital Celebration Health has used the principles of lifestyle medicine to help thousands of patients achieve high performance health. Our approach is very simple: we combine the best of modern medical and surgical techniques with a firm emphasis on lifestyle practices and the need for physicians and patients to form partnerships to achieve optimal outcomes. Every patient leaves our clinic with a detailed plan for how he or she can change lifestyle practices to improve overall health.

This workbook, based on the book *High Performance Health*, has its roots in the successful practice we have built up over the past two decades. The principles and exercises featured in these pages *work*—and even though you may never visit our clinic, you can rest assured that everything you find in this workbook is based on good scientific research and a host of true-life "success stories."

While you can use the workbook on its own, you will benefit most from the process ahead if you use it in tandem with the book. *High Performance Health* cites scores of research studies that will both inform your thinking and underscore crucial concepts, even as it recounts dozens of actual case studies that will serve to inspire your own efforts and suggest possible ways to apply the principles of high performance health.

In my book, *High Performance Health,* I make the strong recommendation that readers keep track of their progress with a journal. The *High Performance Health Workbook* that you have in your hands provides exactly the type of structured journal that will bring the concepts of *High Performance Health* alive in your daily life.

You are about to embark on an exciting journey that has the very real potential to totally reshape for the better your health, your life, and your future—not overnight, not magically, and not without a great deal of effort on your part. But if you really want to pursue and experience the life-changing world of high performance health, you've come to exactly the right place.

And now is exactly the right time to begin.

1 | PROTECT WHAT YOU LOVE

You and I have probably never met, but I'm quite sure I already know one very important thing about you: You love yourself and your family enough to protect your health. How do I know this? Because if you didn't, you wouldn't be using this workbook to personally apply the information and principles detailed in my book, *High Performance Health*. People protect what they love!

So let me start out with a healthy, "Congratulations! You're about to take the next step toward achieving the best life possible by protecting and renewing your health, a precious asset too many of us have taken for granted or simply misunderstood."

And now, let's get down to work!

A TOOL FOR ACCOMPLISHING YOUR DREAMS

What is "high performance health"? It's not merely passive freedom from disease. It doesn't say, "If I feel okay today, that's good enough; I don't have to worry about tomorrow." Instead, it functions as a springboard for achieving a joyous, dynamic, and meaningful life. Your robust health becomes a tool that enables you to accomplish things you've only dreamed about.

High performance health means achieving your best health *now*. It enables you to define your values and set appropriate goals so that you can live every aspect of your life to its highest potential. And it insists that your daily habits have a profound impact on your health and quality of life.

This approach values good health as a precious trust that yields enormous rewards. It sees good health as a network of interrelated values that affect not only your physical health but also your quality of life and spiritual well-being. Six specific values work together to achieve high performance health:

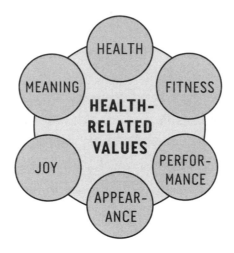

Each of these values—health, fitness, performance, appearance, joy, and meaning—plays a vital role in achieving high performance health as a springboard to high performance living. Each also links health to daily actions.

As you begin to apply to your own life the key concepts from *High Performance Health*, it will be helpful to take stock of where you believe you currently are in each of these six crucial areas. But be honest here! Recognize that Americans tend to grossly overrate their own health. The U.S. Department of Health and Human Services, for example, reports that although more than

90 percent of polled adults consistently rate their health as either "good" or "excellent," the fact is that:

- more than two thirds of Americans are overweight or obese
- about a quarter of men and 20 percent of women still smoke
- less than 25 percent of all adults regularly consume the recommended number of servings of fruits and vegetables
- and only 3 percent of adults observe simple practices that could eliminate 80 percent of heart disease.

How do we explain this discrepancy? It comes down to this—either: (A) someone doesn't understand the question; (B) is not being honest; or (C) pollsters consistently pick out only the American superstars of health.

Unfortunately, the answer is *not* (C).

So again, as you rate yourself in each of the following six areas, try to be as accurate as possible—and as honest as you'd want your doctor to be with you! Circle the number that you believe best represents your current status in that area, from 1 (poor) to 10 (excellent).

SELF-EVALUATION

1. HEALTH

For the purposes of this exercise, "health" means the ability to achieve your optimal physical, mental, and spiritual well-being.

A. My physical health:

1	2	3	4	5	6	7	8	9	10
Poor									Excellent

B. My mental health:

1	2	3	4	5	6	7	8	9	10
Poor									Excellent

C. My spiritual health:

1	2	3	4	5	6	7	8	9	10
Poor									Excellent

D. My overall health:

1	2	3	4	5	6	7	8	9	10
Poor									Excellent

2. FITNESS

"Fitness" here means the capacity to meet or exceed the challenges you face in daily life, whether physical, emotional, social, or spiritual. It includes the adoption of sound health strategies, such as regular medical care, physical activity, nutritional balance, personal connectedness and spiritual well-being.

A. My practice of regular medical care:

1	2	3	4	5	6	7	8	9	10
Poor									Excellent

B. My habits of physical activity:

1	2	3	4	5	6	7	8	9	10
Poor									Excellent

C. My practice of eating regular and nutritionally balanced meals:

1	2	3	4	5	6	7	8	9	10
Poor									Excellent

D. The state of my personal connections to others:

1	2	3	4	5	6	7	8	9	10
Poor									Excellent

E. My spiritual well-being:

1	2	3	4	5	6	7	8	9	10
Poor									Excellent

F. My overall level of fitness:

1	2	3	4	5	6	7	8	9	10
Poor									Excellent

3. PERFORMANCE

Performance is the daily excellence you put into practice to achieve your goals and meet the challenges that life puts in front of you. Performance ultimately rests on daily actions and habits. Performance is what allows you to live in the way you desire.

A. My performance of daily, healthful activities:

1	2	3	4	5	6	7	8	9	10
Poor									Excellent

B. My performance of other healthful habits:

1	2	3	4	5	6	7	8	9	10
Poor									Excellent

C. My overall performance in regard to health issues:

1	2	3	4	5	6	7	8	9	10
Poor									Excellent

4. APPEARANCE

"Appearance" here does not mean physical beauty, but the irresistible attractiveness found in engaging people who always seem full of life. Some of its components include great energy, vitality, and presence.

A. My typical energy level:

1	2	3	4	5	6	7	8	9	10
Poor									Excellent

B. I see myself as alive and vital:

1	2	3	4	5	6	7	8	9	10
Poor									Excellent

C. Wherever I am, my presence is "all there."

1	2	3	4	5	6	7	8	9	10
Poor									Excellent

D. My overall appearance:

1	2	3	4	5	6	7	8	9	10
Poor									Excellent

5. JOY

A powerful relationship exists between your mind and emotions and your body. Good health can stimulate joy, and joy and happiness can nurture good health. To achieve high performance health, it is crucial to create a positive mental environment and find joy.

A. I have created a positive mental environment.

1	2	3	4	5	6	7	8	9	10
Poor									Excellent

B. *My day-to-day experience of joy.*

1	2	3	4	5	6	7	8	9	10
Poor									Excellent

6. MEANING

Living with meaning and purpose is vital to achieving high performance health. Good health can be a source of meaning and purpose, and finding meaning in life contributes in significant ways to overall good health.

A. *My life is filled with meaning.*

1	2	3	4	5	6	7	8	9	10
Poor									Excellent

B. *I know my true purpose in life.*

1	2	3	4	5	6	7	8	9	10
Poor									Excellent

Now that you've finished this opening self-evaluation, how do you feel about the results? Any surprises along the way? Do you feel essentially positive about the current state of your health, or do you sense the need for significant improvement?

Whatever your results, you now have in your possession a *great* basis for beginning (or continuing on) your journey to high performance health. Remember, you have enormous power to be the primary change-agent of your own health. While modern medicine can certainly do wonderful things for you, achieving high performance health depends first and foremost on taking responsibility for yourself.

Take charge in this quest to take back your health! In the exercises and questions that follow, I will not ask you to turn your life upside down, but I *will* ask you to consider very carefully what you can do to improve your health *every day*.

2 | ACHIEVE YOUR BEST HEALTH NOW

A major factor separating the individuals who are able to move forward into high performance health and those who are not is the ability to plan. This workbook is designed to help you craft a personalized plan for achieving high performance health. That plan needs to be both specific *and* geared to the realities of your life—and that includes assessing your current health status, as well as identifying your goals to achieve your best health. After all, if you don't know where you're starting from, then how can you create an effective plan to get you where you want to go?

In chapter 1 you took stock of how well you incorporate the values of high performance health into your own experience. Now it's time to continue your journey by assessing your story.

What has gone on in your life? What *is* going on? The following questions will help you to take a clear-eyed look at where your health is, where you would like it to be, and the factors that are either inhibiting you or standing as assets in your quest for high performance health. By the time you complete the work for this chapter, you should have a baseline picture of your current health and well-being. And just as important, this information will prove very useful in forming a working partnership with your physician as you pursue high performance health.

1. Describe the state of your current health.

_____

_____

_____

2. What health concerns or medical conditions do you have that you believe need your attention?

_____

_____

_____

3. Are you currently under the care of a physician or taking medication for any of these concerns or conditions?

_____

_____

_____

4. What health conditions or medical problems have you had in the past?

_____

_____

_____

5. List any current medications you are taking (prescription, over-the-counter, or nutritional supplements):

_____

_____

_____

6. Have you ever been hospitalized? If so, for what condition? When?

_____

_____

_____

7. Have you ever had surgery? If so, for what condition? When?

_____

_____

_____

8. Do you have allergies to any foods or medicines? Any environmental conditions?

_____

_____

_____

9. Briefly describe your family medical history. Did your mother or father have any chronic conditions, such as heart disease or high blood pressure? Cancer? Did any other members of your immediate family have such medical conditions?

_____

_____

_____

10. Describe your physical activity program (or estimate your current level of regular physical activity). What do you commonly do for exercise? How often do you engage in this activity? How do you feel after your active session is over?

_____

_____

_____

11. Describe any ingrained habits that you believe may promote your health.

_____

_____

_____

12. Describe any ingrained habits that you fear may endanger your health.

_____

_____

_____

13. List the foods that you most commonly eat:

For breakfast

_____

_____

_____

For lunch

_____

_____

_____

For dinner

_____

_____

_____

For snacks

_____

_____

_____

14. Describe your quality of sleep. How many hours of sleep do you normally get each night? Would you describe this sleep as restful or fitful? How do you normally feel when you get up in the morning?

_____

_____

_____

15. Describe the kind of rest you tend to get, outside of sleep. How often do you take breaks throughout the day? What kind of breaks do you take? What kind of rest seems to best recharge your energy level?

_____

_____

_____

16. How often do you take vacations? Describe a typical vacation for you. When was your last vacation? When do you expect to take your next vacation?

_____

_____

_____

17. Do you smoke? If not, have you ever smoked? If so, have you ever tried to quit?

_____

_____

_____

18. Describe your patterns of alcohol consumption.

_____

_____

_____

19. Briefly describe what gives you the most satisfaction:
In your personal life

_____

_____

_____

In your work life

_____

_____

_____

In your relationships

_____

_____

_____

20. Briefly describe what gives you the most dissatisfaction:

In your personal life

_____

_____

_____

In your work life

_____

_____

_____

In your relationships

_____

_____

_____

21. List the biggest areas of stress you face:

In your personal life

_____

_____

_____

At work

_____

_____

_____

In your relationships

_____

_____

_____

22. Describe the nature of your environment:
At home

_____

_____

_____

At work

_____

_____

_____

At church, synagogue, or other frequent destinations

_____

_____

_____

23. What would you say makes you "tick"?

_____

_____

_____

24. Briefly describe your hopes, dreams, and aspirations.

_____

_____

_____

25. What are your health goals?
For the next week

_____

_____

For the next month

_____

_____

For the next year

_____

_____

For the next five years

_____

_____

26. List whatever personal assets you have that you believe will help you to achieve these health goals.

_____

_____

_____

27. List the barriers that you fear will make it more difficult to achieve these health goals.

_____

_____

_____

28. What are your life goals?

For the next week

_____

_____

For the next month

_____

_____

For the next year

_____

_____

For the next five years

_____

_____

For beyond the next five years

_____

_____

29. List the personal assets you have that you believe will help you to achieve these life goals.

_____

_____

30. List the barriers that you fear will make it more difficult to achieve your life goals.

_____

_____

31. Do you tend to look forward to the future with expectation, or with fear and dread? Explain.

_____

_____

_____

The following questions are designed to help you interact with some of the main "teaching points" of chapter 2 from *High Performance Health*. Giving some extended thought to your answers will help you to better understand and apply the principles to follow in the rest of this workbook.

1. Why do you think the ultimate in high performance thinking is to be an optimist? Do you consider yourself an optimist? Would others most likely describe you as an optimist, a realist, or a pessimist? Explain.

_____

_____

_____

_____

_____

2. Describe the connection, love, and support of family and friends that you believe you can expect to receive as you pursue high performance health.

_____

_____

_____

_____

_____

3. How well do you think you are able to give and accept love? Why do you think this is important in achieving high performance health?

_____

_____

_____

4. The major stumbling blocks to achieving high performance health are rooted in negative feelings and attitudes and in a personal sense of unworthiness, not in challenges posed by nutritional changes or an exercise program or other aspects of an action plan. In fact, the main barrier to achieving high performance health comes from within. Deep down, many of us don't think we're worthy of success; we don't consider ourselves "worth the trouble." Do you think you're "worthy of success"? Do you consider yourself "worth the trouble"? Explain.

_____

_____

_____

_____

_____

5. Has a potent feeling of guilt ever kept you from pursuing the best health possible? If so, how can you let go of that guilt? If not, how have you dealt with feelings of guilt?

_____

_____

_____

_____

6. Have you accepted that you're worthy of the gift of life? Explain.

_____

_____

_____

7. Do you believe that you are worthy of the best life you can achieve, simply because God created you? Explain.

_____

_____

_____

8. How can you keep looking forward, planning, and exploring?

_____

_____

_____

_____

9. How can you learn most effectively to live one day at a time?

_____

_____

_____

_____

10. Why does starting down the path of high performance health require faith?

_____

_____

_____

_____

11. What part do planning and persistence play in achieving high performance health?

_____

_____

_____

_____

_____

12. What does it mean to trust yourself in this pursuit of high performance health? How can you best do this?

_____

_____

_____

_____

3 | MASTER THE BASICS

Do you *really* want to improve your health? The men and women who most success-fully jump on the road to high performance health almost always learn how to tap the power of two secrets:

- They master the basics.
- They make change a slow and incremental process.

In this chapter, you will begin to work with these basics—seven key strategies that you can adapt to your personal needs and goals. As you apply them in a gradual, incremental fashion, you will begin to see positive changes take place in your health.

At this stage of your journey to high performance health, remember that most people don't falter because of some big, cosmic issue; they fail because they never figure out how to break up a task into small, easily achievable pieces. The exercises in this chapter are designed to help you avoid that all-too-common error.

SEVEN KEY STRATEGIES FOR HIGH PERFORMANCE HEALTH

When you apply the following seven key strategies for achieving high performance health, you will have begun to master the basics of securing your physical, emotional, and spiritual well-being. Carefully consider each strategy, looking for ways either to incorporate that basic into your life, or how you might improve the ways you apply that key strategy to your own situation.

1. PHYSICAL ACTIVITY

If you were to take only one step to improve your health, that step should be to increase your physical activity. Physical activity keeps all the body's systems tuned for health. In fact, even a moderate amount of physical activity produces marked health benefits. That is why experts at the Centers for Disease Control "urge all Americans to accumulate thirty minutes of moderate physical activity on most, if not all, days."

How many minutes of moderate physical activity do you accumulate on most days? What days seem to be the most difficult for you to grab some exercise? Why?

_____

_____

_____

Note the two key words in the CDC recommendation above: "accumulate" and "moderate." If an activity gets you out of breath, then it's more than what you require.

What type of "moderate" physical activity most appeals to you? What kind are you most likely to pursue? Explain.

_____

_____

_____

_____

What times of day are best suited for you to "accumulate" thirty minutes of moderate physical activity? Are you more likely to engage in such physical activity in a single period, or over several such periods? Explain.

_____

_____

_____

_____

Walking is by far the simplest and most practical way for most people to incorporate increased physical activity into their daily lives. With that in mind, I included a "high performance health walking program" in *High Performance Health* (see pages 217–219 of the book).

Can you envision a walking program as part of your plan for increasing your level of physical activity? Why or why not?

_____

_____

_____

If a walking program appeals to you and you think it might be something you'd like to pursue, what time(s) of day might work best for you? Where might you plan to walk? Where will you walk when the weather turns inclement?

_____

_____

_____

If walking does not appeal to you as a form of good physical exercise, then consider the following. What are the pluses and minuses of each for you in your particular situation?

Cycling (stationary or outdoor)

_____

Jogging

_____

Swimming

_____

Rowing

_____

Dancing

_____

In fact, any exercise that uses the large muscles of your body in a repetitive fashion will work very well. What are some other exercise options that you might find attractive?

_____

_____

_____

How will you find the form of physical activity that is most convenient for you?

_____

_____

_____

How can you most effectively work your way up to accomplishing thirty minutes of this activity on most, if not all, days?

_____

_____

_____

Many people get bored with doing just one physical activity. So what would be some good alternate activities for you?

_____

_____

_____

And remember, you don't have to get all thirty minutes in one session; you can accumulate your physical activity in small increments throughout the day. Which of the following suggestions might work for you?

Walking your dog in the morning
Taking a brisk ten-minute walk at lunch
Taking a pleasant walk with your family in the evening

_____

_____

Increased physical activity will not only lower your risk of heart attack; it's also a great stress reliever.

2. WEIGHT CONTROL

Did you know that more than two-thirds of American adults are either over-weight or obese? The typical adult in the U.S. gains one pound annually. By the time we reach our fifties, the average gain measures more than thirty pounds.

How does your current weight compare to what you weighed in high school or college?

_____

Increased weight increases your risk of developing several chronic diseases, and the more weight you gain, the greater your increased risk. If you've put on thirty pounds since your healthy college days, for example, then you're _four times_ more likely to suffer from heart disease and _twenty to forty times_ more likely to develop diabetes.

Do you have in mind an "ideal weight" for you? If so, what is it? Do you see this as a realistic goal? Why or why not?

_____

_____

_____

Our basic problem? We eat too much and exercise too little. We're tempted by an endless menu of high-calorie, tasty food, and we don't like to get up from the couch. That adds up to a truly toxic environment for weight gain. Nevertheless, it is possible to lose excess weight and keep it off. Those who successfully manage their weight tend to employ four common strategies:

A. They exercise regularly.
B. They are conscious of their daily food choices, eating wisely and controlling their calorie intake.
C. They adopt a long-term mind-set.
D. They find the support of others.

Which of the four preceding strategies is easiest for you to employ? Why? Which of the four is the hardest for you to implement? Why? What can you do this week to improve your application of at least one of these strategies?

_____

_____

_____

_____

_____

While this workbook is intended to give you a good start on the road to weight management, if you would like more help than a workbook can offer, I recommend that you contact Weight Watchers. This fine organization can be found in virtually every big city and through www.WeightWatchers.com.

One very helpful tool you can use in any program to control your weight is a body mass index (BMI) calculator. A good one can be found at www.nhlbisupport.com/bmi/bmicalc.htm.

What is your BMI? What does this number indicate about your current weight? Does it suggest that you need to take any particular action? Explain.

_____

_____

_____

3. FUNDAMENTALS OF NUTRITION

Sound nutrition, along with regular physical activity, can help you significantly reduce your risk of heart disease, stroke, diabetes, high blood pressure, obesity, and more. Perhaps the best single source for reliable information on healthy nutrition is *Dietary Guidelines for Americans*, published by the U.S. government (see the complete guidelines at www.healthierus.gov). The following questions are based on those guidelines:

In a typical day, do you eat a variety of nutrient-dense foods and beverages among the basic food groups? Do you limit your intake of saturated and trans fats (less than 10 percent of calories), cholesterol, added sugars, salt, and alcohol? On the lines, write down the typical foods you eat that don't conform to these guidelines. Does this surprise you in any way?

_____

_____

_____

How do you balance the calories you consume with those you burn?

_____

_____

_____

How well do you emphasize the consumption of certain food groups? On a scale of 1 (completely disagree) to 10 (absolutely agree), rate how closely you conform to the recommended selection of foods for a typical 2,000 calorie diet:

I eat 2 cups of fruit and 2 cups of vegetables daily.

  1   2   3   4   5   6   7   8   9   10

I regularly choose a variety of fruits and vegetables.

1   2   3   4   5   6   7   8   9   10

I eat the equivalent of at least 3 1-ounce servings of whole grains and make at least half of my grain consumption whole grain.

1   2   3   4   5   6   7   8   9   10

I consume 3 cups per day of fat-free or low-fat milk products, or calcium-rich milk product equivalents.

1   2   3   4   5   6   7   8   9   10

I choose fiber-rich foods such as whole-grain breads and cereals, fresh and dried fruit, and beans.

1   2   3   4   5   6   7   8   9   10

I regularly eat breakfast, as I consider it the most fundamental and basic rule of nutrition.

1   2   3   4   5   6   7   8   9   10

I seek the guidance of a professional in helping me to eat properly.

1   2   3   4   5   6   7   8   9   10

For further assistance, you may want to explore some of the helpful nutrition resources that support these dietary guidelines (www.MyPyramid.gov). This Web site, for example, includes a very helpful and flexible planning tool.

4. FUNDAMENTALS OF HYDRATION

You can jump-start your energy and your health through good hydration. Water is a part of every biochemical reaction in the human body and is essential for every aspect of life.

How many 8-ounce glasses of water do you drink in a typical day? How long do you go between drinks of water?

_____

_____

The human body loses three quarts of water on average every day, while physically active people can lose an additional quart. Most people walk around mildly dehydrated, which can cause fatigue and difficulty concentrating.

Have you made it a habit to keep a glass of water on your desk or work area at all times? If not, why not? Remember that it can make an enormous difference in your ability to work long days while minimizing fatigue.

_____

_____

_____

Remember that pure water is best. Avoid beverages that contain sugar, caffeine, and alcohol. Try an experiment for one week. Hydrate for top performance and record the results in the space that follows.

_____

_____

_____

5. SUFFICIENT DAILY REST

Sleep and rest each play a vital role in the healing and restorative processes of the body and contribute significantly to both physical and emotional health. While a great deal of overlap exists between the two, they are not identical. If you fail to get enough sleep and rest, the hustle and stress of your daily life can overload your body's protective defense systems.

At least one recent study has shown that getting seven or eight hours of regular sleep is a strong predictor of good health—yet one out of three American adults does not get adequate sleep.

Describe your typical sleep patterns.

_____

_____

If you get more than six and less than nine hours of sleep—and do not feel sleepy during the day—then your sleep patterns are probably fine.

What kind of caffeinated beverages (coffee, soda pop, etc.) do you drink? How often do you drink caffeinated beverages? Do you avoid them later in the evening?

_____

_____

What time do you normally go to bed? Do you have a "regular" bed time? If not, why not? How could you start going to bed at a more regular time?

_____

_____

_____

Are you overweight? Do you snore significantly or consider your night's sleep restless or intermittent? If so, would you consider being evaluated for sleep apnea or other sleep disorders? Explain.

_____

_____

Do you take sleep medications? If so, did you try adjusting your practices before asking for sleep medication? Explain.

_____

_____

Periods of disciplined rest are a key component of achieving balance, rehabilitation, and recuperation. Even exercise can be a period of rest, to help you maintain balance in life.

Does any form of exercise help you to relax and rest? If so, what is it? How often do you engage in it?

_____

_____

Getting good rest on a daily, weekly, and monthly basis is essential to help you achieve the balance and perspective vital to high performance health. Briefly describe the quality of rest you get:

On a daily basis

_____

_____

On a weekly basis

_____

_____

On a monthly basis

_____

_____

6. CREATING A POSITIVE ENVIRONMENT FOR CHANGE

Stack the deck in your favor by creating a positive environment for change. Focus on three key environmental facets:

A. *Your physical environment*
How easy do your current locales and equipment make it to change your habits?

_____

_____

_____

Do you have plenty of fresh fruits and vegetables available? Are they kept in an easily accessible place, such as on the kitchen counter or washed and ready in the refrigerator? If not, how easy would it be to change this?

_____

_____

Where are some good walking routes near where you live or work? Describe them in the space that follows. Do you have some good walking shoes? If not, where can you acquire some?

_____

_____

Do you have good access to a swimming pool? If so, where is it? Does it require the purchase of a membership? How can you regularly take advantage of it?

_____

_____

Is the activity you want to participate in easily available year-round? If not, how can you overcome this deficiency?

_____

_____

Do you live in a very warm or very cold climate? If so, what kind of indoor places are available for you that can permit you to get regular exercise?

_____

_____

B. *Your social environment*

Whom among your family and friends can you count on for support in your efforts to achieve high performance health? List them here.

_____

_____

_____

_____

What kind of help can you count on from these supportive friends and family? Describe it here.

_____

_____

_____

_____

What can you do, starting today, to develop a supportive health-care team (also see chapter 4)?

_____

_____

C. *Your emotional environment*

Do you believe that you really can get more out of life? Explain.

_____

_____

How can you draw upon your faith to help you achieve high performance health?

_____

_____

What specific things can you do in the next week to build and deepen your confidence that you really can take control of your health?

_____

_____

7. MASTERING THE MIND-SET

A crucial key to achieving high performance health is to change your whole mind-set about health.

How can you frame the way you think about your health to help you achieve the kind of life you want and deserve? What changes in your thinking may have to occur for this to happen?

_____

_____

_____

_____

The most fundamental trait for mastering the correct mind-set for high performance health is to *live in the moment*.

What helps you to focus on today?

_____

_____

_____

How can you avoid spending your time regretting the past?

_____

_____

_____

What most helps you to look to the future with anticipation instead of fear?

_____

_____

_____

What does the phrase "seize the day" mean to you?

_____

_____

How can you most effectively find and use the techniques that work for you to help you live fully and completely in the present?

_____

_____

_____

Choosing the road to high performance health will make all the difference to both your health and your life. Before you proceed further in this workbook, make sure you understand and have begun to incorporate these seven basics into your life. And remember that while you don't have to do all of them at once, you should be aware of all of them. To understand the basics and to begin to incorporate them into your life is an important first step toward achieving high performance health.

4 | BUILD YOUR HIGH PERFORMANCE HEALTH TEAM AND ENVIRONMENT

You will never achieve high performance health if you remain in isolation. You need to build a team that will support and maximize your potential to help you achieve your goal of high performance health. You will also need to maximize your support environment, because it sets the stage for all of your efforts.

And perhaps more important than anything else, for this to work, *you* must captain your own team. You must take charge of the execution, implementation, and follow-through of the plan you are about to develop.

Begin by completing a personal satisfaction inventory. On the following chart, consider the level of satisfaction you receive from each of the individuals, groups, or other personal factors in your life. Rate each factor individually on a scale from 1 (least satisfaction) to 5 (most satisfaction). "NA" means the item does not apply.

PERSONAL SATISFACTION INVENTORY

Family	NA	1	2	3	4	5
Friends	NA	1	2	3	4	5
Spouse	NA	1	2	3	4	5
Children	NA	1	2	3	4	5
Religion	NA	1	2	3	4	5
Sports	NA	1	2	3	4	5
Hobbies	NA	1	2	3	4	5
Work	NA	1	2	3	4	5
Investments	NA	1	2	3	4	5
Community work	NA	1	2	3	4	5

Other (please specify)

_____	NA	1	2	3	4	5
_____	NA	1	2	3	4	5
_____	NA	1	2	3	4	5

• • •

What personal sacrifices have you had to make to achieve success?

_____

_____

_____

List what you consider to be your strongest satisfactions.

_____

_____

_____

From which people or environments do you experience the most support and enjoyment?

_____

_____

Do you need to make any adjustments in the amount of time you spend with these people or environments? If so, what are those adjustments?

_____

_____

BUILDING YOUR HIGH PERFORMANCE TEAM

1. You

This process starts with you. If you are going to benefit from the principles of high performance health, then you are the one who is going to have to take charge. There is no other way.

Do you believe that you are responsible for your own health? Explain. How can you best demonstrate that you are responsible for your own health?

_____

_____

_____

The power of personal encouragement is the cornerstone for building high performance health. You must do what you can to encourage yourself to keep moving down the road of high performance health.

What can you do to encourage yourself to keep going down this road you have already begun? What attitudes or habits of mind might need to change? Which ones need to be strengthened?

_____

_____

_____

_____

Don't fear the hard work of change! It will help you reap the rewards of a purposeful life, one full of meaning.

What changes do you expect will be the hardest for you to make on this journey to high performance health? Why do you think they will be so hard? What can you do to make those changes anyway?

_____

_____

_____

2. Your spouse

If you're married, your spouse can become an indispensable team member. A spouse can provide meaning, calm you down when you feel uptight, and give you an opportunity to both give love and get support. Your spouse is another person with whom you can share both your triumphs and disappointments.

Have you asked your spouse to join your team? If not, why not? If so, what are you asking your spouse to contribute to your team?

_____

_____

_____

Remember, the person who loves you the most wants all the best things for you, including the very best for your health.

What do you see as "the best" for your own health? What does that "best" look like? How have you let your spouse know about this?

_____

_____

_____

Everyone close to you will reap the tremendous benefits from your achieving high performance health. Just don't try to make these changes alone!

3. Family

Your family members can also play important roles on your high performance health team. They probably know you better than anyone else, and they may have unique contributions to make that you won't be able to get anywhere else.

How can you engage your family in your pursuit of high performance health? List several practical ways you can do this.

_____

_____

_____

_____

Which of the following suggestions might be helpful for you to try in your own family? Discuss each one with your family members and see what they say. Write their responses in the space that follows:

Take family exercise outings.

Find ways to improve nutrition for every family member.

Go on a restful vacation or spiritual retreat.

Set a path for your children to emulate; if you engage in regular physical activity, so will your children.

_____

_____

_____

_____

_____

_____

4. Friends

Since friends know you in ways different from your spouse and family, they can provide perspectives that may assist you in both practical and unexpected ways. Friends also provide support that touches and strengthens you in all aspects of your being. Research consistently shows that friends and community have the power to improve your overall health.

Which of your friends do you believe could most effectively serve as members of your high performance health team? Write their names down and describe what contribution you believe each could make.

_____

_____

_____

_____

How do you intend to ask your friends to join your team? Jot down some ideas.

_____

_____

In the space that follows, record when you asked your friends to join your team, as well as their response. This may be helpful later on when you run into some obstacles for which your friends might be able to provide you some assistance.

_____

_____

_____

5. Health-care professionals

Although you are the captain of your own high performance health team, health care professionals should certainly be on that team as well. Consider a few possibilities:

Have you asked your physician to play a role on your team? What can you do to come to the office ready to outline your hopes and health considerations? What do you hope to achieve in the relationship?

_____

_____

_____

If your regular physician does not seem interested in joining your team, will you consider switching to a different physician? If not, why not? If so, what factors will go into choosing another physician?

_____

_____

_____

Have you checked out other sources of medical information and support, such as www.webmd.com? If so, what did you find there? If not, why not?

_____

_____

_____

_____

What qualified nutritionists are available in your area? Have you considered scheduling a one-time consultation with a registered dietician? If not, why not? If so, when will you schedule your consultation?

_____

_____

_____

_____

If you have trouble finding a qualified dietician, you may find the American Dietetic Association to be helpful (www.eatright.org or 1-800-877-1600).

Have you checked out other fine online resources for sound nutritional information? If not, set a time to investigate the following three sites, and write down your discoveries and insights in the space that follows.
www.eatright.org
www.MyPyramid.gov
www.nutrition.gov

_____

_____

_____

What qualified exercise physiologists are available in your area? An exercise physiologist can make sure your exercise program is safe and effective and fits your interests and environment. If you don't know how to locate a qualified exercise physiologist, try the following resources, and then write down your discoveries in the space that follows.
Local hospital wellness centers
YMCAs
A quality fitness center
The trade association IHRSA (International Health, Racquet, and Sportsclub Association)

_____

_____

_____

Have you considered having a conversation about your health goals with your local pharmacist? Make sure you understand the health purposes of any medications you are taking, as well as their appropriate uses. Ask your pharmacist for a frank evaluation of any supplements you are taking, and write down your discoveries in the space that follows.

_____

_____

_____

6. *Other supportive partnerships*

The primary principle here is to make sure you don't try to go on this journey alone. All of us need help here! And the strengthening of relationships alone is worth the effort of seeking out team members.

Who do you know that has goals similar to your own? Who could be a like-minded partner for your team? Write down some possible names in the space that follows, and identify a date by when you will contact these individuals to inquire about becoming a member of your team.

_____

_____

_____

What self-help groups or affinity groups do you know of that could be willing and useful members of your team? Write them down.

_____

_____

_____

Who might be an effective and willing mentor for you on this journey? Write down the names of a few prospective mentors.

_____

_____

_____

Do you have a spiritual mentor who might be able to function well on your team? Remember the profound medical connections between mind, body, and spirit. Write down the name of such an individual, and then set a time when you will ask the person to join your team.

_____

_____

_____

No doubt there are people all around you who would be willing and able to serve effectively as members on your high performance health team. Remember, these needn't be "formal" relationships. You're just looking for interested men and women who can help you succeed on this important journey you've begun.

CONSTRUCTING A HIGH PERFORMANCE HEALTH ENVIRONMENT

If you're like most people, you need an environment that encourages you to be your best—and *you* need to take responsibility for creating it. This environment includes both physical surroundings and more intangible factors.

1. Create a supportive physical environment
Where will your primary physical activity take place?

_____

_____

If you plan to walk, have you mapped out walking trails or routes of various distances? If so, write down the names and distances of a few trails. If not, why not?

_____

_____

_____

_____

What inclement weather alternatives have you identified? Write them down.

_____

_____

What equipment have you acquired to make your exercise both enjoyable and effective?

_____

_____

What times and places have you arranged to meet others to participate with you?

_____

_____

Have you stocked your pantry, refrigerator, and freezer with healthy foods? If so, list a few of them in the space that follows. If not, why not?

_____

_____

What two or three different fresh fruits do you have available for snacking?

_____

_____

_____

In the space that follows, create a grocery list that will help you to stick with your new choices and avoid temptations.

_____

_____

_____

_____

_____

_____

_____

Have you emptied your pantry of nutritionally-empty snacks and drinks? If so, list the items you have eliminated. If not, what's keeping you from eliminating these unhealthy sources of extra calories?

_____

_____

How can you keep yourself from getting too hungry between meals? Write down a few ideas to try.

_____

_____

Have you considered joining a support group? If so, what group are you joining or looking to join? If not, why not?

_____

_____

2. Find a "third place."

Your journey toward high performance health will be greatly enhanced if you have "a third place" beyond home and work—a place where you will be surrounded by caring people who share the same interests or mission that you do. This might be a church or faith community, a health club, a social or fraternal club, a garden club, a volunteer group, a book club, or a hobby group.

If you already have "a third place," write it down, and indicate what benefit you hope to gain from it in regard to your high performance health team.

_____

_____

If you do not yet have "a third place," in the space that follows identify some possible candidates, and then indicate when you will investigate each one to see whether it would be a good fit.

_____

_____

_____

3. Volunteer

The unselfish act of doing good for others also yields important benefits for your own health.

Where have you volunteered in the past? Would you consider doing this again? Why or why not?

_____

_____

What "new" volunteer opportunities appeal to you? Where can you find out more information about volunteering in these areas?

_____

_____

What reasons in the past have you given for not volunteering? What are some good answers to these objections?

_____

_____

When can you realistically begin (or continue) some new volunteer work? Write down the date, and then write out your plans for volunteering.

_____

_____

4. Create a positive mental environment
What mind-set for high performance health have you created? Describe it.

_____

_____

How do you plan on connecting with other people?

_____

_____

What preparations have you made to forgive people who have hurt you?

_____

_____

Describe how you have forgiven yourself and affirmed that you are worthy.

_____

_____

What can you do to make sure you voyage forward, and not drift backward?

_____

_____

Identify at least three people you want on your team and three changes in your environment that you are going to make.

_____

_____

5 | TRANSFORM YOUR LIFE THROUGH HIGH PERFORMANCE THINKING

Using your mind as a powerful ally to frame issues in your life in a more positive and achievable light is what I call high performance thinking. I believe you can accomplish whatever you can dream—and the essentials of high performance thinking can help you to achieve those dreams.

Performance is simply the ability to do those things in your daily life that bring you meaning, happiness, and fulfillment. Performance enables you to meet life's challenges without losing your equilibrium or core confidence. It permits you to keep moving toward your goals, regardless of the challenges you face.

High performance thinking draws on the powerful connections between your mind, body, and spirit. This chapter will help you to tap these vital mind-body-spirit connections through applying eight aspects of high performance thinking—thus enabling you to transform your mind-set into a powerful ally for high performance health and high performance living.

THE EIGHT ESSENTIALS OF HIGH PERFORMANCE THINKING

1. PASSION

Passion is the fuel that drives performance. It implies not only energy, but a deep set of values and caring about a topic. Passion allows you to go beyond the expected norms and accomplish the incredible. In essence, it allows you to get *more* out of life.

What are you passionate about?

_____

_____

_____

What do you think you could be passionate about?

_____

_____

What would you like to be more passionate about?

_____

_____

How passionate are you about your health?

_____

_____

How does your passion about your health translate into specific action?

_____

_____

_____

_____

2. TRUST

Trust allows you to let go of guilt and live for today. It keeps you "in the moment" and has three main components:

A. Trust in yourself.

You must believe that you are capable of making positive changes that will improve your life. Believing you can accomplish a worthy goal is fundamental to accomplishing that goal.

Do you believe that you are capable of making positive changes that will improve your life? If so, how is this belief shaping your actions? If not, why not?

_____

_____

_____

What small steps are you taking to build your trust in yourself? List some of them in the space that follows.

_____

_____

_____

B. *Trust in others.*

Trust in others is fundamental to learning and improving. Being trustworthy in relationships and trusting in others to provide the same support frees you up to let go of certain worries . . . and even to fly.

How easy is it for you to trust others?

_____

_____

Why do you think it's important for you to trust others in this journey toward high performance health?

_____

_____

What steps can you take to increase your trust in others, especially regarding your pursuit of high performance health?

_____

_____

C. *Trust in God.*

Trust in God enables you to sense order and consistency in the world. Trusting that God the Creator is ever present and ever working within you and through you enables you to live in the moment and seize the day. Trust in God makes it easier to rid yourself of anxiety so that you can focus on the tasks necessary to achieving high performance health and more meaningful living.

Do you trust in God? If so, how? If not, why not?

_____

_____

How can trust in God help you to "seize the day"?

_____

_____

How do you think trust in God tends to decrease anxiety? Does this occur in your own life? Explain.

_____

_____

_____

Would you like to increase your level of trust in God? If so, how might you be able to do this? If not, why not?

_____

_____

_____

3. COURAGE

It takes courage to carefully assess both your strengths and your weaknesses, looking for areas of needed change that promise to improve your life and health.

What do you see as your greatest strengths in your pursuit of high performance health?

_____

_____

What do you see as your greatest weaknesses in your pursuit of high performance health?

_____

_____

What areas of your life appear to be most in need of change if you are to achieve high performance health? How will courage be necessary to make these changes?

_____

_____

What would you like to try first? Write it down in the space that follows. And remember, it takes courage to go out and walk five or ten minutes if you have been totally sedentary.

_____

_____

How can you best break your identified goals into small steps? Describe this process in the space that follows.

_____

_____

_____

_____

How can you best give yourself credit for having the courage to make a needed change?

_____

_____

_____

    As you exercise the courage to make whatever changes you think are necessary, you can be sure that the desired improvements will come.

4. DISCIPLINE

Every high performance individual I've ever met has developed a keen sense of discipline. Appropriate structure, provided through discipline, enables these people to make daily progress. Discipline frees up space, time, and resources—not just for work on goals, but for other important activities, people, and interests.

Write down in the space that follows your key assessments, plans, daily progress, and reflections.

_____

_____

_____

_____

_____

In the space that follows, "make an appointment" for your next exercise session.

_____

_____

What structure and discipline seems to work best for you? Describe it in the space that follows.

_____

_____

_____

List three ways that you are going to establish positive routines in your daily life.

_____

_____

_____

5. FOCUS

The best way to benefit from your discipline is to sharply focus on the key tasks or objectives you need to accomplish each day. Focus is the ability to order tasks into priorities and then to devote single-minded attention to each task. Focus helps you conquer mundane distractions. Focus turns the light of discipline into the laser of achievement.

What are the key tasks or objectives that you need to accomplish today? How about for tomorrow? For the rest of this week?
Today:

_____

_____

Tomorrow:

_____

_____

Rest of the week:

_____

_____

_____

_____

How would you prioritize the tasks and objectives you listed above? What comes first, second, third, etc.?

_____

_____

_____

_____

_____

_____

_____

What are the most consistent distractions you face on a daily basis? List them in the space that follows.

_____

_____

_____

_____

How can you best overcome these distractions? What is your plan of attack to overcome each one? (Example: if answering emails is a distraction that takes you away from your key tasks, you could choose to answer them only at certain times each day.)

_____

_____

_____

_____

6. CONSISTENCY

A wise consistency is vital to accomplishing every important goal. Consistency is the key to reaping long-term health benefits and to turning your health into a springboard for high achievement. Routines are a fundamental way to achieve consistency. Routine provides stability and balance and can help you focus on what is important.

How consistent do you think you tend to be? Would others agree with this assessment? Explain.

_____

_____

_____

Describe in the space that follows a few of your most important and common routines.

_____

_____

_____

How do these routines help you to accomplish your most important tasks and goals?

_____

_____

_____

_____

For the next week, record what works and doesn't work for you. Then use that information to help you craft and modify your own routines. Remember, this will lead to consistency—and ultimately, to higher performance.

_____

_____

_____

_____

_____

_____

_____

_____

_____

_____

_____

7. HAPPINESS

Since finding true joy is essential to good health, happiness is worth pursuing. Remember that whatever brings you joy also brings you good health.

What makes you happy?

_____

_____

_____

What tends to steal your happiness?

_____

_____

_____

How can you better focus on the issues that bring you joy and jettison the distractions that keep you from it?

_____

_____

_____

List three aspects of your life in which you find true happiness and ways that you will work to increase that level of happiness.

_____

_____

_____

8. PRAYER

In prayer you open yourself to communication with God. You consciously get yourself in a place where you can live in God's presence. I see prayer—which involves both speaking and listening—as an organizing principle and a source of comfort that links you to a sense of a larger mission and order in the universe, controlled and watched over by the Creator.

How do you see prayer? How would you describe it?

_____

_____

How often do you pray? How would you describe your prayer life?

_____

_____

What does it mean to you to "live in God's presence"? How might this lead to better health?

_____

_____

_____

In your experience, how does prayer involve speaking?

_____

_____

In your experience, how does prayer involve listening?

_____

_____

How does prayer link you to a larger sense of mission and order in the universe?

_____

_____

_____

How does prayer give you comfort?

_____

_____

How can you make prayer a larger part of your life, especially in connection with your pursuit of high performance health?

_____

_____

_____

6 | REVITALIZE YOUR HEALTH THROUGH EMOTIONAL WELL-BEING

Each of us is a complex being with an exuberant emotional life inextricably woven together with a complex physical existence. We ignore the interconnections between our emotions and our bodies at our peril.

Beyond that, if we do not examine and understand how to channel, control, and modify our emotions, then we make it much more difficult for ourselves to achieve high performance health. So we must learn to "talk" with ourselves, look within, understand our emotional responses and reactions, and examine how some of those responses may block health and well-being and how others may support and nourish health.

In this chapter we will focus on:

- several major emotions that are key to achieving your best health now
- the triggers for these emotions
- the emotion-driven behaviors that can either impede or improve your ability to achieve high performance health.

WHO AND WHAT IS IN CONTROL?

You have an enormous opportunity to control your health and your own path in life. You really do! But to experience this in all its fullness, you first have to turn your emotional life into a powerful ally.

Do you consider your emotions an ally, or an enemy, in your efforts to achieve high performance health? Explain.

_____

_____

_____

Did you know that the emotional links to pain (and how you understand those links) may make all the difference between whether that pain is tolerable and manageable or whether it becomes a major distraction from what is really important to you? In almost _any_ circumstance, how you feel about what's happening can either distract you or serve as a powerful force to help you move forward. Since emotions can serve as both challenges and opportunities, we'll look at both types.

In my book _High Performance Health_ I develop how the interconnectedness of the emotions and the physical body works to promote either health or encourage disease (see pages 96–98). Here I want to help you to do two things: work to modify or heal the emotional responses or emotion-triggered behaviors that are blocking you (the challenges); and to draw on those that can strengthen you (the opportunities).

THE CHALLENGES

1. STRESS

Broadly speaking, stress is any force that requires a response or change, whether emotional or physiological. While a certain amount of stress helps you to focus on achieving your goals, it becomes destructive or negative when it overwhelms your psychological and physiological capacity to constructively deal with it, neutralize it, or even benefit from it. The way in which you handle the many inevitable stressors in your life in large measure determines whether the impact on your health and well-being will be neutral, negative, or positive.

PERSONAL STRESS INVENTORY

A. How much job-related stress do you usually have?

Very little   Moderate amount   Quite a bit   Extreme amount

B. How much negative job-related stress do you usually experience?

Very little   Moderate amount   Quite a bit   Extreme amount

C. How well do you think you cope with your job-related stress?

Poorly   Fairly well   Moderately well   Very well

D. How much stress do you experience in your personal life?

Very little   Moderate amount   Quite a bit   Extreme amount

E. How much negative stress do you experience in your personal life?

Very little   Moderate amount   Quite a bit   Extreme amount

F. How well do you think you cope with your personal stress?

Poorly   Fairly well   Moderately well   Very well

G. Do you have any symptoms that may relate to your stress?

Yes   No

If yes, please list them:

_____

_____

Where do you experience the most stress in your life?

_____

_____

What kind of stress is it? How would you characterize it?

_____

_____

In what areas of your life can you work to reduce harmful stress?

_____

_____

Describe how you think you might be able to begin to cope more effectively with stress.

_____

_____

How do you use regular physical activity to manage your stress?

_____

_____

Name some ways you could use regular physical activity to better manage your stress:

_____

_____

Consider a few other ways to reduce stress as well.

Since regretting the past or fearing the future serves only to pile on the stress, how can you better learn to live in the present? In other words, what can you do—starting today—to seize the day?

_____

_____

Look for ways to avoid adding a negative emotional overlay to your stress. What things do you tend to worry about over which you have no control? List them in the space that follows.

_____

_____

_____

_____

How can you best benefit from "the Serenity Prayer," which says, "God, grant me the serenity to accept the things I cannot change, the courage to change the things I can, and the wisdom to know the difference."?

_____

_____

_____

What does it mean to you to "get out of your own way"? How can this help you relieve stress?

_____

_____

_____

Describe your plan to deal with stress.

_____

_____

_____

_____

What specific techniques or strategies help you to best manage and release your stress? Describe them.

_____

_____

_____

Do you ever leave stress "free-floating"? How can you deal with "free-floating" stress?

_____

_____

_____

2. ANGER

The kind of anger that endangers your health usually arises in response to day-to-day irritations, slights, and vexations. You may use other terms to describe it—blaming, cynicism, impatience, hostility, resentment, hate—but it's still anger, and it can still kill. Failure to control a constant undercurrent of anger jeopardizes your health.

Two simple techniques can help you avoid or defuse anger:

A. *Ask, "Can I change it? Is it in my control?"*
If the answer is no, then the only thing you *can* control is your response.

What fairly insignificant matters tend to spark anger in you? How can you better release your irritation with these things?

_____

_____

For one week, keep a log of every time something triggers an angry response in you. Write down those incidents in the space that follows. Then after you've cooled off, evaluate your anger—where it came from, what it accomplished, the damage it did. How can becoming better aware of your anger help you to defuse it?

_____

_____

_____

_____

_____

B. *Give yourself a personal time-out.*

Clearly communicate your need to cool down and your intention to take a personal time-out until you can calmly discuss the issue and rationally respond to it.

Write down how you would tell someone that you need to take a time-out. Then practice saying it before you need to use it.

_____

_____

_____

_____

Learning to better trust others often helps to reduce anger. What can you do to increase your level of trust in others (especially those who tend to trigger angry responses in you)?

_____

_____

The next time you grow angry with someone, try to put yourself in his or her shoes for a moment. Try to imagine what might have prompted this person to act as he or she did. In other words, try a little empathy. Then write down what you learned.

_____

_____

_____

_____

Is it generally easy for you to forgive someone who has injured you? If not, why not? Does your unwillingness to forgive the person actually "pay back" the person for the injury? Explain.

_____

_____

_____

_____

3. ANXIETY AND DEPRESSION

Anxiety typically involves exaggerated worry and tension, often about everyday matters. Depression can involve feelings of worthlessness, meaninglessness, hopelessness, emptiness, or deep anxiety. Fatigue often accompanies both.

Do you often feel anxious? If so, what usually causes these feelings?

_____

_____

_____

How do you typically deal with your feelings of anxiety?

_____

_____

Would you say that you seldom or frequently battle with depression?

_____

_____

When you feel anxious or depressed, are you usually involved in some kind of regular physical activity? What kind of connection do you think there could be here?

_____

_____

_____

Do you think losing weight might help you battle anxiety or depression? Explain.

_____

_____

Take some time to set a few realistic goals about dealing with your anxiety or depression, and list some specific actions you can take to accomplish them, along with a realistic timeline.

_____

_____

_____

_____

_____

_____

When was the last time you consulted your physician and asked for a thorough evaluation?

_____

_____

How can you best work with your physician to create a balanced therapeutic plan for yourself?

_____

_____

4. PAIN AND GRIEF

No one lives in this world without getting hurt. No one avoids losses, whether in relationships or in that final loss, death. Loss not only wounds our spirits, it also stresses our bodies. Anger, fear, guilt, and feelings of isolation and hopelessness may mount.

Do you agree that pain is one of the prices we pay for being full and whole human beings? Explain.

_____

_____

How can you learn from pain to turn it to a positive purpose?

_____

_____

Describe how you give yourself space and permission to grieve and to cry.

_____

_____

To whom can you reach out for support?

_____

_____

_____

How can going for a walk or doing some other physical activity help you to cope with the pain?

_____

_____

5. DENIAL

Anxiety, fear, guilt, depression, and other motivators often prompt us to deny unpleasant truths—and denial is a terribly dangerous emotional response to life. We all tend to indulge in the Tomorrow Promise: "I'll start planning for high performance health tomorrow."

What small step toward change can you make today that will help you to stop fooling yourself?

_____

_____

_____

In what ways have you not yet achieved all you need out of life?

_____

_____

_____

How can you do better?

_____

_____

You really can get out of this deadly pattern of denial—and start experiencing the good health that you want and deserve—by making a conscientious effort to make small, positive changes in your daily life.

List any emotional challenges you have and outline some ways you are going to work to overcome them.

_____

_____

_____

THE OPPORTUNITIES

1. LOVE

The capacity to love and be loved is a cornerstone value for high performance health and high performance living. When you love, you give of the best of yourself. When you are loved unconditionally—as God loves you—you are freed to stretch and keep growing. You open yourself to great joy and happiness, as well as to vulnerability, pain, and grief. In short, you give yourself the possibility of becoming a fully realized human being.

What does "love" mean to you? Why is it important for high performance health?

_____

_____

How do you generally try to show others your love for them?

_____

_____

How do you generally try to receive the love others have for you?

_____

_____

Do you believe that God loves you unconditionally? If not, why not? If so, what does this love look like, and how does It affect the way you live?

_____

_____

Would you say that you are on your way to becoming "a fully realized human being"? Explain.

_____

_____

_____

_____

2. CONNECTEDNESS AND COMMUNITY

A key component of achieving high performance health is to "reach out and touch someone." Healthy human connections and growing community are vital to your success.

How are you nurturing your connectedness and sense of community with others?

_____

_____

What kind of time and effort do you take to establish close connections with others?

_____

_____

Who would you name as the people closest to you? What makes them close? Do you wish they were closer still? Explain.

_____

_____

_____

3. SPIRITUALITY

Carefully cultivating and nurturing your spirit will yield multiple and important health benefits that will spill over into virtually every aspect of your life.

What things best cultivate and nurture your own spirit?

_____

_____

What things tend to crush and injure your spirit?

_____

_____

Do others tend to consider you a "spiritual" person? If so, why? If not, why not?

_____

_____

Do you have a desire to deepen your own spirituality? If so, how do you plan to do so? If not, why not?

_____

_____

4. PURPOSE

Since life is a journey and not a destination, the quest for purpose is dynamic. A sense of purpose gives backbone and a sense of transcendence to life.

Do you believe that if a person has not discovered something worth dying for, then he or she isn't fit to live? Explain.

_____

_____

What do you see as your own purpose for living?

_____

_____

_____

What could you do to increase a sense of purpose in your life?

_____

_____

_____

Who do you know personally that exhibits a real sense of purpose? What do you admire most about this person? How do you think you could become more like him or her?

_____

_____

_____

_____

5. HOPE

Hope is one of the touchstones of emotional health and has much in common with optimism and vision. It looks forward, works forward, and focuses on living. And it enjoys the life it lives.

How would you describe hope?

_____

_____

Do you consider yourself a hopeful person? Explain.

_____

_____

How can you make hope your ally in your pursuit of high performance health?

_____

_____

_____

6. FORGIVENESS

Practicing true forgiveness—despite its difficulty—is a powerful way to revitalize your health and well-being. Letting go of injury and insult and relaxing your grip on internal wounds is like unlocking the chains that have shackled you to old injuries. Just as important is seeking forgiveness (and letting go of guilt) when you have hurt someone else.

What do you think it means to forgive someone?

_____

_____

Would you describe yourself as a forgiving person? Explain.

_____

_____

Why does it often seem so difficult to forgive someone who has hurt you?

_____

_____

Does "letting go of insult and injury" mean that you let an offender "off the hook"? Explain.

_____

_____

Do you think extending forgiveness to someone who has hurt you could help your own pursuit of high performance health? Explain.

_____

_____

Who do you need to forgive? What has kept you from forgiving this person? Who has been most hurt by your refusal to forgive, the guilty person or you?

_____

_____

Whose forgiveness do you need for some hurt that you have caused? What stops you from seeking this individual's forgiveness?

_____

_____

List several emotional opportunities you have to improve your health and describe how you are going to take advantage of them.

_____

_____

_____

Many of the issues we have discussed about healing your own emotions to revitalize your health can be passed on to your children. Name several ways in which your own emotional healing can benefit your children.

_____

_____

_____

List some ways you can participate in your own healing process and a few specific actions you can take to enhance them.

_____

_____

_____

_____

7 | STOP TO REST AND HEAL

Rest and healing *literally* keep you alive. Rest provides time for your body to heal from the daily damage inflicted by the stresses of living, even as it rejuvenates your energy and spirit.

What kind of rest does your body most seem to need?

_____

_____

How do you provide time for your body to rest?

_____

_____

Does your best rest involve exercise? Remember, sometimes you must expend energy to gain energy. What kind of exercise allows you to rest?

_____

_____

How disciplined are you about taking regular periods of rest throughout the day? Describe your basic rest habits.

_____

_____

_____

_____

ACTIVE REST

Active rest has five components:

1. REPAIR

Every day, every cell in your body suffers from one thousand to one million molecular "lesions." This damage needs to be repaired. Left unrepaired, such damage can lead to cancer, various autoimmune disorders, and even accelerate the aging progress.

How can you effectively reduce your exposure to toxic environments?

_____

_____

What destructive habits do you have (such as overeating or smoking) that you need to change?

_____

_____

Remember that rest helps your body repair its structures at all levels.

2. SLEEP

Most adults need seven to eight hours of sleep each night for optimal functioning.

How many hours of sleep do you normally get?

_____

Do you believe you could benefit from enhancing your sleeping patterns?

_____

If you answered "yes" to the question above, try some of the following proven strategies to enhance your sleeping patterns.

A. Adopt positive lifestyle activities that enhance sleep.
What kind of regular physical activity do you get during the day?

_____

_____

Do you know the importance of avoiding exercise right before bedtime? What other times during the day could you exercise instead?

_____

_____

Describe a diet that you would consider nutritious and balanced. Do you eat such a diet?

_____

_____

_____

_____

Do you avoid spicy food and caffeinated beverages for dinner or within two hours of bedtime?

_____

Do you avoid alcohol late at night?

_____

B. *Keep to a sleep schedule.*
What time do you normally go to bed? Do you have a regular bedtime schedule that you like to keep? If not, why not?

_____

_____

What have you done to make sleep a habit?

_____

_____

How quickly do you normally fall asleep at night?

_____

_____

What can you do to arise at your scheduled time, even if you didn't fall asleep quickly when you went to bed?

_____

_____

C. Control sleep-preventing stimuli.

It's important to use your bedroom for sleep and not for activities incompatible with sleeping, such as eating, playing loud music, or watching television.

Do you often eat in bed?

_____

What kind of music best helps you to fall asleep?

_____

_____

Do you have a television in your bedroom? If so, have you considered taking it out? Explain.

_____

_____

What room temperature helps you to fall asleep and stay asleep? Can you adjust the thermostat to the optimal temperature?

_____

_____

_____

Is your bedroom either too light or too dark for you to get restful sleep? If so, what can you do to change the environment?

_____

_____

_____

D. *Learn relaxation techniques.*
Have you tried a relaxation program on CD?

_____

_____

_____

Have you ever tried a technique like the following: *Lie in a comfortable position, visualize the progressive relaxation of your body, starting with your toes. Intentionally relax them, letting them sink comfortably into the bed each time you breathe out. Move smoothly up to your lower and upper legs, your hips, your torso. Push intrusive thoughts away; focus on breathing and relaxing?*
Try it and then record your experience in the space that follows.

_____

_____

_____

_____

E. Consider cognitive therapy.

Cognitive therapy can help some individuals replace mental blocks with realistic expectations.

What fears or beliefs do you have that may interfere with your ability to sleep?

_____

_____

3. RETREAT

Occasional retreats away from the hustle and bustle of "ordinary" life are crucial for maintaining proper rest in your life.

How have you disciplined yourself to take regular periods away from the stresses of your current situation?

_____

_____

What room in your schedule have you made for longer periods of retreat and escape?

_____

_____

Use the following space to make a basic plan for a regular one-day or longer retreat to help you regroup, reenergize, refocus, and relax.

_____

_____

_____

_____

When in the next year can you take an extended vacation?

_____

_____

How can you make this extended vacation a time of spiritual and physical rejuvenation?

_____

_____

_____

What types of retreats most effectively restore your body and soul?

_____

_____

_____

4. RELAX

Relaxation may be the critical element that separates champions from the merely great. Staying on an even keel, never getting too high or too low, is critical to performance.

What present concerns make you mentally or physically tense? Identify them in the space that follows, and then consciously think about letting them go.

_____

_____

_____

_____

_____

How can you practice keeping an even keel?

_____

_____

_____

How can you best work with your body and not against it?

_____

_____

_____

5. ACTIVELY RECOVER

"Active recovery" assists your body in getting rid of toxic waste products, whether they be physical or emotional. This allows healing to take place.

How intentional have you been about getting your necessary rest?

_____

_____

_____

What may you need to do—what may need to change—for you to get the rest that you require? What intentional changes should you consider?

_____

_____

_____

HEALING

Continuous healing is at the core of high performance health. Let's look at several common medical conditions—skip the ones that don't pertain to you—and briefly suggest a few things you can do to promote active healing.

1. HEART DISEASE

What kind of regular physical activity are you engaging in to counter this condition?

_____

_____

Describe your nutritional patterns.

_____

_____

Are you working to maintain a healthy body weight?

_____

If you have been a smoker, are you quitting, or have you quit?

_____

How are you attempting to control your blood pressure? (See helpful resources at www.americanheart.org and www.nhlbi.nih.gov.)

_____

_____

2. CANCER

We could eliminate an astonishing *70 percent* of all cancers in the United States if people stopped smoking, maintained a healthy weight, stayed out of the sun during peak sun exposure, and followed a few other basic practices.

What kind of ongoing, caring relationship with your doctor(s) have you established?

_____

_____

What kind of regular exercise program have you adopted?

_____

_____

Have you altered your diet to get proper nutrition (see www.cancer.org for helpful suggestions here)?

_____

_____

3. OBESITY

Obesity triples the risk of heart disease and increases the risk of diabetes by forty times. That means losing weight is not merely an appearance issue; it's a health issue. Weight loss programs that work incorporate all four key strategies.

A. A sound approach to nutrition

Are you getting the nutrients necessary for health while reducing energy intake?

_____

_____

_____

B. Regular physical activity

Are you engaging in moderate activity on most, if not all, days? Remember that this helps maintain lean muscle and boosts your metabolism and energy.

_____

_____

C. Adopting a long-term mind-set

What is your long-term strategy for losing weight?

_____

_____

_____

D. The support of others

Who have you enlisted to help you in your efforts to reduce your weight (www.weightwatchers.com has some helpful suggestions)?

_____

_____

_____

4. HIGH BLOOD PRESSURE

High blood pressure is a major risk factor for both heart disease and stroke.

Are you getting regular exercise? Are you walking thirty minutes on most, if not all, days?

_____

Have you lowered the amount of sodium (salt) in your diet by eating less processed foods and more natural fruits, vegetables, and grains?

_____

What efforts have you made to lose weight—even five or ten pounds?

_____

_____

5. ARTHRITIS

Paying attention early in life to weight management and getting regular physical activity can help you avoid arthritis in later years.

When you are injured, what attention do you pay to injury rehabilitation and healing?

_____

_____

What supportive medication do you take?

_____

_____

Describe your current level of physical activity.

_____

_____

How are you handling weight management?

_____

_____

(www.arthritis.org can provide some other helpful information.)

6. SMOKING

Smoking is the leading cause of preventable death in the United States. Yes, it's hard to stop smoking and quitting may take many tries—but the payoff is worth it.

What medications have you used to try to stop smoking?

_____

_____

What structured programs have you investigated in your efforts to stop smoking?

_____

_____

What online smoking cessation support groups have you looked into?

_____

_____

7. SPIRITUAL HEALING

True healing comes only from *both* physical and spiritual healing.

To whom have you reached out for support (family and friends, clergy, fellow sufferers)?

_____

_____

What spiritual resources are available to you to help you connect with others and with God?

_____

_____

Now that you have considered at length the crucial issues of rest and healing, take a few minutes to chart out how you will achieve disciplined periods of rest:

Daily:

_____

_____

Weekly:

_____

_____

Monthly:

_____

_____

Finally, list any specific health conditions you have, and describe how you are going to reframe your actions to reclaim your good health.

_____

_____

_____

_____

_____

8 | OVERCOME THE SEVEN MAIN BARRIERS TO HIGH PERFORMANCE HEALTH

What keeps many people from enjoying high performance health? They struggle with at least one of the seven main barriers to high performance health. So in this penultimate chapter, we'll identify each one and suggest some ways to overcome them.

BARRIER 1: FAILURE TO FRAME ISSUES PROPERLY

Your primary task is to think of your health as a high performance tool rather than as simple freedom from disease. Consider it a dynamic way to get more out of life. Beware of three common errors here.

1. SHORT-TERM THINKING

Quick-fix weight loss schemes simply don't work. The key is to accept that effective weight loss is a slow, progressive process—about one pound per week, using portion control and regular exercise.

What "quick-fix" weight loss schemes have you tried? What results did you get?

_____

_____

Why is it so hard in this culture to accept that effective weight loss is a slow, progressive process?

_____

_____

What can you do to help yourself accept the fact that a weight loss of about a pound a week is not only adequate, but excellent?

_____

_____

2. NOT TAKING PERSONAL RESPONSIBILITY FOR YOUR HEALTH.

Your health is not your doctor's responsibility; it's yours. Positive lifestyle practices should be your frontline strategy for promoting health. The best outcome is always achieved through a true partnership between you and your physician.

Who is responsible for your health?

_____

What positive lifestyle changes have you made to promote your own health?

_____

_____

_____

_____

What kind of partnership have you formed with your physician?

_____

_____

_____

3. BELIEVING MOST DISEASE CANNOT BE PREVENTED.

Not all disease can be avoided, but focusing on proven, preventive measures can help you reduce your risks and establish a firm foundation for achieving high performance health.

What kind of effect can you have on your most pressing health concerns?

_____

_____

How can you properly frame your health issue?

_____

_____

BARRIER 2: ALL-OR-NOTHING THINKING

Positive change is most likely to occur if you think of such change as an incremental process. The key is to *gradually* integrate positive health behaviors into your life.

What is your basic health goal?

_____

_____

What small subgoals can help you to achieve this overall health goal?

_____

_____

If your goal is to walk a mile a day, what smaller subgoals could lead up to that goal?

_____

_____

If your overall goal is to start eating right, how can you gradually integrate more fruits, vegetables, and whole grains into your meals and snacks?

_____

_____

What will you do when you stumble a bit? How will you react when you temporarily "fall off the wagon"?

_____

_____

How will these small changes you make fit into the normal fabric of your life?

_____

_____

_____

BARRIER 3: POOR PLANNING AND PREPARATION

Poor planning and a failure to prepare adequately prevent many people from reaching their health goals. So whatever important changes you want to make to enable you to achieve your health goals, make sure you have planned well and adequately prepared for them.

If you travel often, how can you arrange to choose hotels that have fitness centers? Thirty minutes on a stationary bike can do wonders!

_____

_____

_____

How can you most effectively remember to pack your walking or running shoes when you go on a trip?

_____

_____

_____

Take a few moments to describe what would be an enjoyable, active vacation for you:

_____

_____

_____

_____

How can you avoid environments that seem full of temptation?

_____

_____

How will you plan and prepare to make these changes?

_____

_____

BARRIER 4: NOT LIVING IN THE PRESENT

Regrets about the past and fears about the future prevent many people from achieving high performance health. Focusing on the present enables you to cope with today without carrying the emotional baggage of past regrets and future fears.

What specific regrets about the past tend to haunt you? What can you do to keep them in the past, where they belong?

_____

_____

What specific fears about the future tend to worry you? How can you refuse to let these fears negatively color your present?

_____

_____

What can you do _today_ to fully live in and enjoy the present?

_____

_____

BARRIER 5: NOT RECOGNIZING YOUR THREE AGES

Everyone has three "ages": chronological, physiological, and spiritual. While you can do nothing about your chronological age (except to work to keep living!), you can do plenty about the other two.

A. *Chronological age (your age in years since your birth)*
    The great baseball legend Satchel Paige once said, "Age is a case of mind

over matter. If you don't mind, it don't matter." In fact, aging has multiple benefits, including a deeper appreciation for life and a more profound ability to love.

How much does your chronological age matter to you?

_____

_____

What benefits to aging have you experienced so far?

_____

_____

Do you appreciate life now more than you used to? Explain.

_____

_____

How has aging expanded your ability to love?

_____

_____

B. Physiological age (the functioning age of your organs and muscles)

Satchel Paige also used to say, "How old would you be if you didn't know how old you were?" Did you know that regular physical activity can alter the physiological age of your body's cardiovascular system? In addition, getting appropriate nutrition and other healthful lifestyle practices can positively alter your body's other systems.

Answer Satchel's question: How old would you be if you didn't know how old you were?

_____

_____

Do you expect that your current patterns of physical activity and nutrition are positively altering your body's critical systems? Explain.

_____

_____

C. Spiritual age (emotional age of your spirit)

It's worth remembering this quote one more time: "Work like you don't need the money. Love like you've never been hurt. Dance like nobody's watching." What a gift it is to be around optimistic and energetic individuals! It's inspiring to see their willingness to take on new challenges and try new things throughout their lives.

Do you work like you don't need the money?

_____

_____

Do you love like you've never been hurt?

_____

_____

Do you dance like nobody's watching?

_____

Do you consider yourself optimistic and energetic? Do others say how much they enjoy being around you?

_____

_____

Are you willing to take on new challenges, regardless of advancing age?

_____

_____

What specific things can you do to enhance your spiritual age?

_____

_____

BARRIER 6: FAILURE TO RECOGNIZE YOU HAVE THE POWER TO CHANGE YOUR HEALTH

Repeatedly we have noted how regular physical activity lowers the risk of virtually every chronic disease. In addition, consuming five or more servings of fruits and vegetables each day and eating at least three one-ounce servings of whole grains is associated with lower risk of many cancers, heart disease, high blood pressure, and diabetes. You have the power to change your life for the better!

Is your current level of physical activity likely to lower the risk of your contracting a disease? Explain.

_____

_____

Are your current eating habits likely to lower the risk of your contracting a disease? Explain.

_____

_____

How are you demonstrating through your beliefs and actions that you have the power to improve your health and enhance your life?

_____

_____

BARRIER 7: THINKING THAT CHANGE IS EASY

Change is never easy. In fact, it's almost always difficult. *But you can do it*—you really can achieve high performance health. But this requires both dedication and hard work. It may be helpful to ponder how many people work through several stages to arrive at helpful change.

Stage One: Precontemplation. Before someone is ready to change, the mere thought of change can seem daunting. You may hear them say, "Get off my back!" But there are constructive ways to encourage change.

What most helped you to start considering the benefits of some difficult change?

_____

_____

How can you use what you learned from your own experience to encourage someone else to follow a healthier life path?

_____

_____

What does your experience show that you should avoid in trying to encourage others to make healthy changes?

_____

_____

Stage Two: Contemplation. When a pondered change seems less hurtful than the status quo, a person begins to think about what that change would mean. He or she may say, "I want to stop feeling so stuck." You can counter their anxiety with expressions of excitement and helpful knowledge.

What benefits of a proposed change most encouraged you to actually make the change?

_____

_____

_____

What kind of statements and expressions from others prompted you to move along the new path?

_____

_____

Stage Three: Preparation. People at this stage begin to make plans to accommodate the contemplated change. They're getting ready to take the plunge and so say things like, "I'll start tomorrow." They use this time to develop an effective plan of action.

How did you feel at this stage? Or are you at this stage right now?

_____

_____

Why is it a good idea to make plans in the face of anticipated change?

_____

_____

Stage Four: Action. There comes a time when you need to take the first step and begin that first leg of the journey: "Here I go!" At this stage you continue to learn helpful methods and secure the support you need.

What was the most significant action you took to begin your journey toward high performance health?

_____

_____

What methods and sources of support are you continuing to collect as you move forward?

_____

_____

Stage Five: Maintenance. Long after the excitement of beginning a new venture fades, you must continue to find ways to forge ahead. "Keep going forward!" is the rallying cry at this stage. It's helpful to create a plan for dealing with slips and lapses in order to achieve long-term success.

If you've been at this for a while, what is the most difficult thing for you to do to keep moving ahead toward high performance health?

_____

_____

_____

Describe your plan for dealing with slips and lapses in order to achieve long-term success.

_____

_____

_____

_____

Stage Six: Termination. Although all temptations may not disappear, you can still achieve lasting, positive change. You, too, can cry, "Home free!"

What temptations continue to give you the most problems?

_____

_____

What successes can you celebrate already that point to your achieving lasting, positive change?

_____

_____

What one specific change would you like to make in your life? Write it down in the space that follows.

_____

_____

Develop a doable strategy for overcoming the seven barriers to this change.

_____

_____

What will you do to make the commitment and accomplish the hard work to make this change a permanent part of your life?

_____

_____

9 | USE HIGH PERFORMANCE HEALTH AS A SPRINGBOARD TO HIGH PERFORMANCE LIVING

High performance living is the ability to consistently perform at your best to meet whatever challenges confront you. In this chapter you will apply the following nine principles of high performance health to enhance your entire life.

1. ENERGY

While high performance *health* provides abundant energy, the goal of high performance *living* is to use that energy wisely.

How would you describe your current levels of energy? Are they increasing?

_____

_____

Where do you tend to spend your energy?

_____

_____

_____

How well do you focus on issues critical to your success?

_____

_____

How do you handle distractions?

_____

_____

How much energy do you spend on the people and activities that are important to you?

_____

_____

_____

If you would like to spend more of your energy on the people and activities that mean the most to you, what needs to change in your life?

_____

_____

What plan do you have for making the changes you identified in the question above?

_____

_____

2. FOCUS

Focus allows you to perform and achieve at your maximum—and the ability to focus comes from practice and discipline. Further, breaking down big goals into smaller, specific tasks allows you to focus and so achieve superior results.

How have your personal practices and disciplines allowed you to achieve better focus?

_____

_____

How could you improve at breaking your big goals down into smaller, specific tasks?

_____

_____

What "big goal" do you currently have that could benefit from being broken down into smaller, more specific tasks?

_____

Make a stab at breaking the "big goal" identified above into smaller, more specific tasks.

_____

_____

_____

_____

3. GOAL SETTING, PLANNING, AND ORGANIZATION

Goal setting is the first step in the planning and organization process. Taking time to plan saves time later and can free up time for family and activities you value.

Where do you want to be five years from now?

_____

_____

What direction do you want to pursue in your career?

_____

_____

What are the important goals and aspirations you would like to achieve in your life?

_____

_____

What are your three most important overall goals?

_____

_____

_____

_____

Name three of your intermediate goals. These take from one week to six months to complete and point to some milestone or establish some deadline (for example, perhaps you want to lose ten pounds over the next three months, or establish a regular exercise program in the next six months).

What are your three most important daily goals?

What plans do you have for accomplishing your long-term, intermediate, and daily goals?

_____

_____

_____

_____

What plan do you have for evaluating your long-term, intermediate, and daily goals? How do you plan to revise them, if necessary?

_____

_____

_____

_____

_____

_____

When you break your bigger tasks into small ones that can be accomplished and evaluated on a daily basis, even a huge task becomes manageable—and the job gets done well.

4. COMMITMENT

Commitment means giving 100 percent of yourself to achieve some important task or objective. When you give yourself wholly to high performance health, you gain joy, energy, and freedom. Committing yourself to the purposes and people you most value will be richly rewarding.

How committed are you to achieving high performance health?

_____

_____

_____

What kind of joy, energy, and freedom have you already experienced as you pursue high performance health?

_____

_____

What kind of rewards do you look forward to as you continue on the journey of high performance health?

_____

_____

_____

What will it take for you to remain committed to this journey that you've begun?

_____

_____

_____

5. PERSPECTIVE

Occasionally you have to step back and look at the entire process of high performance health, as if you were standing outside. This helps you to stay on an even keel when you hit those stretches where nothing seems to be moving forward and nothing seems to be going your way. Perspective gives you the freedom to let the problems go and keep moving forward.

How does long-term thinking nourish good perspective?

_____

_____

_____

How would you rate your current perspective?

1	2	3	4	5	6	7	8	9	10
Poor									Excellent

If your perspective needs a boost, what are some good ways for you to step back and look at the entire process?

_____

_____

What problems or obstacles have you already surmounted in your pursuit of high performance health? How can recalling these victories help to broaden your perspective and strengthen your resolve to keep moving forward?

_____

_____

What friends or family may be able to help you clarify your goals or get you through tough times?

_____

_____

How can you best listen to others and honor their points of view?

_____

_____

6. POSITIVE HABITS AND THE PURSUIT OF EXCELLENCE

Habits are repetitive actions performed until they become so routine that you rarely think about them.

What negative habits do you have that you need to get rid of?

_____

_____

What positive habits do you need to establish or strengthen?

_____

_____

How can you best foster habits that support your stated goals?

_____

_____

The goal here is to develop good habits and engrain them so deeply in your life that they lead inevitably to excellence.

7. LEADERSHIP

Remember that you are the captain of your own life. Viewing yourself as a leader helps you to effectively use high performance principles for both yourself and those around you.

What kind of leader do you consider yourself to be, especially in your pursuit of high performance health?

_____

_____

Name several instances of how you lead by example in the ways you work with and relate to others.

_____

_____

_____

How can you become a better leader, especially as you pursue high performance health?

_____

_____

Where is your leadership taking both you and those who follow you?

_____

_____

8. RESPONSIBILITY

To get the most out of your health and your life, you must assume responsibility for both. While you can't always control your circumstances, you can always take responsibility for how you respond to them. There is no magic substitute for taking daily responsibility for your own choices and actions as you work to achieve high performance health and use it as a springboard to high performance living.

In what situations do you feel most tempted to refuse to take responsibility for your choices and actions?

_____

_____

How can you overcome the temptation noted above?

_____

_____

What is involved in taking daily responsibility for the way you respond to whatever life throws at you?

_____

_____

_____

9. RELATIONSHIPS

Supportive, valued relationships are central to achieving high performance health. What we love, we will protect. And what we love is worth living fully for.

What relationships mean the most to you, and why?

_____

_____

_____

_____

How do you plan to protect these relationships?

_____

_____

_____

_____

How can you most fully live for those you love?

_____

_____

_____

_____

10 | FIND YOUR PURPOSE AND EMBRACE YOUR DESTINY

The final, and most important, step in achieving high performance health is to connect it to the things you most deeply value. Embracing your destiny can also be the most rewarding part of the journey, because it leads to the wellsprings of purpose and meaning.

In this final chapter I invite you to think about some of the qualities that help you build bridges to discovering (or rediscovering) the people, purposes, and pursuits that can give your life greater meaning.

1. LIVING INTENTIONALLY

Living intentionally means that you pay close attention to the daily fabric of your life. It's hard, it takes discipline, and it demands that you step back to make plans and set priorities. Living intentionally also means that you choose where you focus your energy and creativity.

How do you keep track of "the daily fabric of your life"? What methods do you use to pay close attention to the everyday events of your life?

_____

_____

List your top ten priorities in life. How do your plans reflect these priorities?

_____

_____

_____

_____

_____

_____

_____

_____

What demands most of your energy? Is this where you really want to focus your energy? Explain.

_____

_____

2. LOVE AND INTIMACY

Love is the cornerstone of health and an essential component for finding your purpose and embracing your destiny. I like Dr. Scott Peck's definition of love: "the will to extend one's self for the purpose of nurturing one's own or another's spiritual growth." Such love requires attention and fuels courage, takes risks and makes commitments, and provides the conviction to confront others when they have fallen off the path.

If love is the cornerstone of health, is it a cornerstone and hallmark of your life? Explain.

_____

_____

How have you extended yourself for the purpose of nurturing your own or another's spiritual growth?

_____

_____

Why does your love require attention? How does it fuel courage?

_____

_____

In what ways does your love take risks? What kind of commitments has it made?

_____

_____

Does your love have the conviction to confront others (in love!) when they have fallen off the path to health? If so, how does it do so?

_____

_____

_____

3. FAITH AND TRUST

Faith and trust are critical to achieving good health and to finding meaning and purpose in life. No wonder the apostle Paul singled out faith, along with hope and love, as the three keys to living an abundant life (see 1 Corinthians 13).

Are you convinced that this world has an order and a purpose, and that your life also has a purpose? Explain.

_____

_____

How have you searched for your life's purpose? What have you discovered on this search?

_____

_____

Why is it necessary to have faith in yourself as well as faith in God?

_____

_____

How does faith give you the courage to find your purpose and embrace your destiny?

_____

_____

Do you believe you are living out your life's purpose? Explain.

_____

_____

4. COMPASSION

Compassion joins us in community. Compassion helps us to help one another. Compassion calls us out of ourselves and enables us to offer ourselves to others.

What does "compassion" mean to you?

_____

_____

Why is compassion necessary for building community?

_____

_____

Do you consider yourself a compassionate person? Explain.

_____

_____

Describe the most compassionate person you know. What do you most admire about this person? What would you most like to emulate? Why?

_____

_____

_____

How is compassion calling you out of yourself and enabling you to offer yourself to others?

_____

_____

_____

5. ACCEPTANCE

Some individuals stumble on the path to achieving high performance health and high performance living because they do not feel they deserve such gifts. You must learn to accept that you are worthy of forgiveness. Accepting forgiveness enables you to move forward. Acceptance means that you believe you are worthy of the joy that comes from a disciplined and thoughtful pursuit of improved health and purpose.

Do you ever feel guilty that your own choices and behaviors have contributed to the challenging situations you face? If so, how do you respond to this sense of guilt?

_____

_____

Do you believe that you are worthy of enjoying high performance health? Why or why not?

_____

_____

How can you help others to believe that they are accepted and worthy of the joy of a sound mind and body?

_____

_____

6. SPIRITUALITY

You must not neglect your spirit if you want to enhance your whole life. If you want a life rich in purpose and meaning, then you need spiritual sustenance every bit as much as you need food.

What spiritual activities tend to feed your soul?

_____

_____

_____

_____

Describe how you have experimented in trying to discover a life of purpose
and meaning.

_____

_____

Describe your most precious passions and your dreams. How have you
given yourself permission to pursue them?

_____

_____

Why is it important that you make your own discoveries in the spiritual
realm?

_____

_____

7. JOY

Joy is not mere pleasure, but a deep-seated sense of well-being that comes from finding fulfillment and meaning in life.

What burdens will you have to lay down in order to open the door to joy?

_____

_____

_____

How have you dealt with resentment?

_____

_____

How do you overcome envy and other joy-killers?

_____

_____

Describe how you practice living in the present.

_____

_____

How are you trying to find your own path to joy?

_____

_____

How have you been surprised by joy?

_____

_____

8. GRACE

In one sense, grace is the collective unconscious that empowers you to do good. It frees you from fear and fills you with praise and joy. It releases you from fears about yourself, allowing you to act with power.

How would you describe grace?

_____

_____

How does grace release you from fears about yourself?

_____

_____

How does grace allow you to act with power?

_____

_____

What discoveries have you made about how grace works in your life?

_____

_____

9. GROWTH AND MATURITY

It takes courage to grow and mature, because venturing into the unknown can be scary. It is possible to leave a current, unsatisfactory situation only if you have the courage and conviction that you can create, prompt, or work toward positive change.

Do you feel that you are currently growing and maturing? Explain.

_____

_____

What scary "unknown" do you wish to venture into? What makes it scary?

_____

_____

What positive change do you most want to work toward?

_____

_____

What do you envision your life looking like in five years? Ten? Twenty?

_____

_____

_____

_____

10. ALONENESS VERSUS LONELINESS

Some aspects of pursuing purpose and meaning are deeply personal, requiring that you spend some time alone. As you grapple with many issues in quiet dialogue with your own thoughts and spirit, you needn't feel isolated or deserted. You can be alone without feeling lonely.

What elements of pursuing your true purpose and meaning feel deeply personal to you?

_____

_____

In what settings can you most effectively have significant dialogues with your own thoughts and spirit?

_____

_____

Describe a time when you were alone but didn't feel lonely.

_____

_____

Plan a time this week when you can be alone with your thoughts. Sketch out a rough "agenda" to guide your meditation.

_____

_____

What insight or memorable concept do you most value from a recent time of contemplation and meditation?

_____

_____

_____

11. TELLING YOUR STORY

A valuable part of creating purpose and meaning in your life comes from sharing your story. Your example and your wisdom can touch and inspire others in ways you may not imagine. By telling your story, you give of yourself.

What most excites you about telling your story? What most unnerves you? Why?

_____

_____

Describe a time when, by sharing part of your story, you encouraged or helped someone else. What happened?

_____

_____

What parts of your story seem most profound to you? What parts still seem most mysterious? Why?

_____

_____

At what points in your story do elements of meaning and purpose most bubble up through the narrative? What do these parts of your story tell you about your purpose?

_____

_____

_____

_____

Do you believe there is a higher power that ultimately provides meaning and purpose to all of life? Explain.

_____

_____

How can the values or qualities discussed in this chapter help you to achieve the goals you laid out in chapter 9?

_____

_____

_____

_____

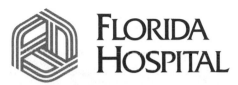

FLORIDA HOSPITAL

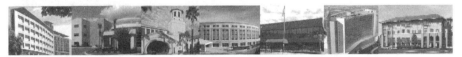

AMERICA'S TRUSTED LEADER FOR HEALTH AND HEALING

For nearly one hundred years the mission of Florida Hospital has been to help our patients, guests and friends achieve whole-person health and healing. With seven hospital campuses and sixteen walk-in medical centers, Florida Hospital cares for over one million patients every year.

Over a decade ago Florida Hospital began working with the Disney Corporation to create a groundbreaking facility that would showcase the model of healthcare for the twenty-first century and stay on the cutting edge of medical technology as it develops. Working with a team of medical experts, industry leaders, and healthcare futurists, we designed and built a whole-person health hospital named Celebration Health located in Disney's town of Celebration, Florida. Since opening its doors in 1997, Celebration Health has been awarded the *Premier Patient Services Innovator Award* as "The Model for Healthcare Delivery in the 21st Century."

When Dr. Lydia Parmele, the first female physician in the state of Florida, and her medical team opened our first healthcare facility in 1908, their goal was to create a healing environment where they not only treated illness, but also provided the support and education necessary to help patients achieve whole-person health mentally, physically, spiritually, emotionally, and socially.

The lifestyle advocated by our founders remains central to all we do at Florida Hospital. We teach patients how to reduce the risk of disease through healthy lifestyle choices, encouraging the use of natural remedies such as fresh air, sunshine, water, rest, nutrition, exercise, outlook, faith, and interpersonal relationships.

Today, Florida Hospital:

- Ranks number one in the nation for inpatient admissions by the American Hospital Association.
- Is the largest provider of Medicare services in the country.
- Ranks number one in the nation for number of heart procedures performed each year. MSNBC named Florida Hospital "America's Heart Hospital".
- Operates many nationally recognized centers of excellence including Cardiology, Cancer, Orthopedics, Neurology & Neurosurgery, Digestive Disorders and Minimally Invasive Surgery.
- Is one of the "Top 10 Best Places in the Country to have a Baby" according to *Fit Pregnancy* magazine.

For more information about Florida Hospital and our other whole-person health products, including books, music, videos, conferences, seminars, and other resources, please contact us at:

Florida Hospital Publishing
683 Winyah Drive, Orlando, FL 32803
Phone: 407-303-7711   Fax: 407-303-1818
Email: healthproducts@flhosp.org
www.FloridaHospital.com   www.CreationHealth.com

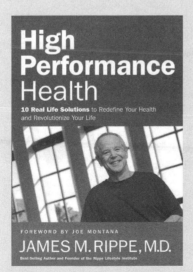

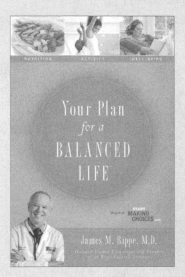